COPING WITH DEMENTIA

A GUIDE TO DEMENTIA CARE

BY

DR. LIMA GARETH

COPYRIGHT

No part of this book should be copied, reproduced without the author's permission @ 2024 "COPING WITH DEMENTIA

TABLE OF CONTENT

Chapter 1 5
Understanding Your Diagnosis 5
   What is Dementia? 5
   Defining Dementia and its Types 8
   How Dementia Affects Daily Life 11
   What to Expect After Diagnosis 14
   Managing Feelings of Uncertainty and Anxiety 17
   Adapting Daily Routines and Activities 19
Chapter 2 23
Treatment Options and Relief Strategies 23
   Herbal Remedies and Supplements 23
   Exploring Natural Remedies for Dementia
   Symptoms 25
   Herbal Supplements and Their Potential
   Benefits 28
   Safety Considerations and Potential Interactions 30
Chapter 3 33
   The Role of Nutrition in Dementia Management 33
   Foods and Nutrients That Support Cognitive
   Health 35
   Developing a Dementia-Friendly Diet Plan 37
Chapter 4 40
Physical Activity and Exercise 40
   Exercise as a Non-Pharmacological Treatment
   for Dementia 40
   Crafting a Diet Plan for Someone with Dementia 42

    Types of Exercises Beneficial for Cognitive
    Function 44
    Implementing an Exercise Routine for
    Individuals with Dementia 47
Chapter 5 51
Mindfulness and Relaxation Techniques 51
    Mindfulness Meditation and its Impact on
    Cognitive Function 54
    Incorporating Relaxation Techniques into Daily
    Care 57
Chapter 6 62
Cognitive Stimulation Activities..............................62
    Engaging Activities to Support Brain Health and
    Function 62
    Cognitive Stimulation Therapy Approaches 65
    Creating Stimulating Environments for.............70
    Individuals with Dementia 70
Chapter 7 75
Understanding Common Symptoms of Dementia .75
    Memory Loss and Cognitive Decline................75
    Behavioral and Psychological Symptoms 79
    Physical Challenges and Health Considerations81
Chapter 8 84
Strategies for Managing Symptoms at Home 84
    Creating a Supportive Environment 84
    Practical Tips for Daily Living 87
    Seeking Professional Assistance and Supportive
    Services 90

Chapter 1

Understanding Your Diagnosis

What is Dementia?

Dementia is a complex syndrome characterized by a decline in cognitive abilities that interferes with daily life. It's not a specific disease but rather a term used to describe a range of symptoms associated with a decline in memory or other thinking skills severe enough to reduce a person's ability to perform everyday activities. Alzheimer's disease is the most common cause of dementia, accounting for 60-80% of cases. Other types include vascular dementia, Lewy body dementia, and frontotemporal dementia.

The hallmark symptom of dementia is memory loss, particularly short-term memory loss. However, it also affects other cognitive functions such as language, attention, problem-solving, and visual perception. As the condition progresses, individuals may struggle to recognize familiar faces or places, have difficulty communicating, and experience changes in mood or behavior.

Alzheimer's disease, the most prevalent form of dementia, is characterized by the accumulation of abnormal proteins in the brain, including beta-amyloid plaques and tau tangles, which disrupt communication between brain cells and lead to their eventual death. Vascular dementia, on the other hand, is caused by reduced blood flow to the brain, often due to stroke or other vascular conditions, resulting in damage to brain tissue. Lewy body dementia is associated with abnormal protein deposits called Lewy bodies, while frontotemporal dementia affects the frontal and temporal lobes of the brain, leading to changes in personality, behavior, and language.

Dementia is a progressive condition, meaning symptoms worsen over time. Early diagnosis is crucial for accessing appropriate treatment and support services, as well as for planning for future care needs. While there is currently no cure for most forms of dementia, various medications and therapies can help manage symptoms and improve quality of life for both individuals with dementia and their caregivers.

Caring for someone with dementia can be challenging and emotionally taxing. As the condition advances, individuals may require increasing levels of assistance with daily activities such as bathing, dressing, and eating. Caregivers often face significant stress and may experience feelings of guilt, frustration, and isolation. It's essential for caregivers to prioritize self-care and seek support from healthcare professionals, support groups, and other caregivers to prevent burnout and maintain their own well-being.

In addition to medical treatments, there are many practical strategies that can help individuals with dementia remain independent and engaged in daily life for as long as possible. These may include modifying the home environment to reduce safety risks, implementing memory aids such as calendars and reminder systems, and encouraging participation in stimulating activities such as puzzles, games, and social outings.

Public awareness and understanding of dementia are crucial for reducing stigma and ensuring that individuals affected by the condition receive the support and respect they deserve. Education campaigns aimed at raising awareness about dementia risk factors, warning signs, and available resources can help promote early detection and access to care. Inclusive communities that prioritize the needs of individuals with dementia and their caregivers can also play a significant role in fostering social inclusion and enhancing quality of life for those affected by the condition.

Defining Dementia and its Types

The term "dementia" refers to a group of neurological conditions marked by a deterioration in cognitive abilities that makes it difficult to carry out daily tasks. There are various varieties of dementia, each with unique characteristics, causes, and progressions, while Alzheimer's disease is the most prevalent type. For proper diagnosis, care, and support for patients and their carers, it is essential to comprehend these many kinds.

1.Alzheimer's Disease: Alzheimer's disease accounts for the majority of dementia cases, estimated at around 60-70%. It is characterized by the accumulation of abnormal protein deposits in the brain, such as beta-amyloid plaques and tau tangles. These deposits lead to the death of nerve cells and the progressive deterioration of cognitive abilities, particularly memory, thinking, and reasoning skills. Alzheimer's disease typically begins with mild memory impairment and gradually worsens over time, affecting language, judgment, and personality. While the exact cause is unknown, genetic and environmental factors are thought to play a role.

2. Vascular Dementia:Vascular dementia is the second most common type of dementia, accounting for around 20% of cases. It occurs due to reduced blood flow to the brain, often as a result of strokes, small vessel disease, or other vascular issues. The symptoms of vascular dementia can vary depending on the location and severity of the brain damage but often include difficulties with executive function, attention, and speed of thought. Risk factors for vascular dementia include hypertension, diabetes, smoking, and high cholesterol levels.

3.Lewy Body Dementia (LBD):Lewy body dementia is characterized by the presence of abnormal protein deposits called Lewy bodies in the brain. These deposits disrupt the normal functioning of brain cells, leading to a range of cognitive and motor symptoms. Hallucinations, fluctuations in alertness and attention, movement disorders resembling Parkinson's disease, and REM sleep behavior disorder are common features of LBD. It is the third most common cause of dementia, accounting for around 5-10% of cases.

4.Frontotemporal Dementia (FTD): Frontotemporal dementia primarily affects the frontal and temporal lobes of the brain, leading to changes in behavior, personality, and language. Unlike Alzheimer's disease, which primarily affects memory, FTD often presents with early behavioral and personality changes, such as disinhibition, apathy, or socially inappropriate behavior. Language difficulties, including difficulty finding the right words or understanding language, may also occur in some cases of FTD. FTD is relatively rare compared to other types of dementia, accounting for around 5% of cases.

5. Mixed Dementia:Mixed dementia refers to a combination of two or more types of dementia, often Alzheimer's disease and vascular dementia. It can present with overlapping symptoms and may have a more rapid progression compared to single-type dementias. Mixed dementia is common in older adults and poses unique challenges for diagnosis and management.

How Dementia Affects Daily Life

The neurological condition known as dementia is a degenerative condition that causes several difficulties in all aspects of daily living. The effect of dementia on memory, communication, routine, behavior, and relationships is evident from the minute a person gets up until they go to bed. Envision awakening to a world that seems even more foreign. Memory loss makes simple things like brushing your teeth or preparing breakfast difficult. People feel vulnerable and disoriented when the familiar landmarks of their own house become less clear. Trust and security, which once grounded their everyday lives, may be undermined when they forget where they put important things or even find it difficult to identify loved ones.

Communication, the cornerstone of human connection, becomes a labyrinth of frustration and misunderstanding. Words slip through fingers like grains of sand as individuals struggle to articulate their thoughts or grasp the meaning of conversations around them. The inability to express oneself or comprehend others breeds isolation, turning once vibrant social interactions into solitary islands adrift in a sea of confusion.

Daily routines, once the scaffolding of stability, crumble under the weight of cognitive decline. Tasks that were once second nature—a morning cup of coffee, a stroll around the neighborhood, or balancing a checkbook—now require Herculean effort or fall by the wayside entirely. As routines unravel, so too does a sense of purpose and autonomy, leaving individuals adrift in a sea of uncertainty.

Behavioral changes further complicate an already tangled landscape. Mood swings, agitation, or aggression may erupt like storm clouds on a seemingly clear day, leaving both individuals with dementia and their caregivers reeling in their wake. Repetitive behaviors, like pacing or rearranging objects, offer temporary respite from the fog of confusion but can quickly become exhausting for all involved.

The toll on relationships is perhaps the most profound. Loved ones watch helplessly as the person they once knew slips further away, replaced by a shadow of their former self. Conversations that once flowed effortlessly now falter, punctuated by long pauses and misunderstandings. The bonds that once held families together are strained as caregivers grapple with the dual burdens of grief and responsibility.

The need for constant care and supervision adds another layer of complexity to an already overwhelming situation. As dementia progresses, individuals may become increasingly dependent on others for even the most basic tasks of daily living. Caregivers, often family members, shoulder the immense responsibility of tending to their loved one's needs while juggling their own obligations and emotions.

Financial strain compounds the already heavy burden of caregiving. The cost of medical care, home modifications, and specialized assistance can quickly deplete savings and strain familial relationships. Difficult decisions about long-term care options loom on the horizon, forcing families to confront their own mortality and the limitations of their resources.

Amidst the chaos and uncertainty, moments of clarity and connection offer glimmers of hope. A shared laugh, a tender touch, or a familiar melody can momentarily bridge the gap between past and present, reminding both individuals with dementia and their caregivers of the love that endures even in the face of adversity.

In the face of such formidable challenges, resilience becomes not just a virtue but a lifeline. Accessing support services, building a network of allies, and embracing the power of community can help individuals and families navigate the uncharted waters of dementia with grace and dignity. Though the road ahead may be long and arduous, each step taken in solidarity is a testament to the strength of the human spirit in the face of adversity.

What to Expect After Diagnosis

After someone is told they have dementia, a lot of things start to change. It's like going on a journey with twists and turns, but there are some things we can expect along the way.

First, it's important to know that dementia is something that gets worse over time. This means that the things someone can do, like remembering stuff or thinking clearly, might not be the same as before. But everyone's journey with dementia is different, and some people might experience changes faster or slower than others.

When someone gets diagnosed with dementia, they work with doctors and other experts to make a plan. This plan helps them figure out the best ways to manage the symptoms and make life easier. It's like having a roadmap to guide them through the journey ahead.

Feeling all sorts of emotions is normal after getting a dementia diagnosis. It's okay to feel sad, mad, scared, or confused. Talking to friends, family, or people who understand what they're going through can help them cope with these feelings.

As dementia progresses, the person might find it harder to do things they used to do easily. They might forget things more often, feel confused, or have trouble with everyday tasks like cooking or getting dressed. It's important for the people around them to be patient and understanding, and to help out when needed.

Making the home safe and comfortable becomes really important as dementia gets worse. Simple changes like adding grab bars in the bathroom or removing things that could cause tripping accidents can make a big difference. Caregivers also need to pay attention to the person's emotional needs and encourage them to stay active and engaged in activities they enjoy.

Taking care of someone with dementia can be a big job, and caregivers need to remember to take care of themselves too. It's okay to ask for help from family, friends, or professionals, and to take breaks when needed.

As dementia progresses, the person might need more help with everyday things like eating, moving around, and taking care of themselves. In some cases, they might need to move to a special place where they can get the extra help they need.

Lastly, it's important for everyone involved to learn as much as they can about dementia and the support services available. This knowledge can help them make informed decisions and find the best ways to support the person with dementia throughout their journey.

So, getting a dementia diagnosis is like starting a new chapter in life's book. It's not always easy, but with love, patience, and support, people with dementia and their families can navigate this journey together.

Managing Feelings of Uncertainty and Anxiety

Coping with uncertainty and anxiety in dementia can be tough, whether you're the person with dementia or their caregiver. But there are ways to handle those feelings and make things a little easier.

First, it's important to understand what dementia is and how it affects people. Learning about the condition can help you know what to expect and feel more prepared for the challenges ahead. Knowledge can help ease fears and make things less scary.

Talking openly about feelings is another important step. If you're the one with dementia, sharing your thoughts and worries with someone you trust can help you feel supported and understood. And if you're a caregiver, being honest and listening to the person with dementia can provide reassurance and comfort.

Establishing routines and sticking to them can also help. Having a daily schedule with regular meal times, bedtime routines, and familiar activities can create a sense of stability and predictability. Knowing what to expect each day can reduce anxiety and make things feel more manageable.

Creating a comforting environment is key. Surrounding yourself with familiar objects, photos, and mementos can provide a sense of continuity and connection to the past. Caregivers can also help by staying calm, patient, and understanding during challenging moments.

Finding activities that bring joy and meaning can lift spirits and distract from worries. Whether it's listening to music, working on puzzles, or spending time outdoors, engaging in enjoyable activities can boost mood and provide a sense of accomplishment.

Staying connected with others is important for both the person with dementia and their caregiver.

Spending time with friends, family, and community members can provide emotional support and companionship. Joining support groups or participating in dementia-friendly programs can also help combat feelings of isolation.

Practicing relaxation techniques can help calm the mind and reduce stress. Deep breathing exercises, meditation, and yoga can promote relaxation and improve mood. Even simple activities like going for a walk or doing gentle exercises can help clear the mind and ease tension.

Finally, don't hesitate to seek professional help if needed. Mental health professionals can provide coping strategies, emotional support, and practical guidance for managing feelings of uncertainty and anxiety in dementia. Support groups can also offer a sense of community and understanding.

Adapting Daily Routines and Activities

Adapting daily routines and activities for someone with dementia is like customizing a game to make it more enjoyable and manageable. Here are some simple strategies to help make each day smoother and more enjoyable:

1. Stick to Simple Routines: Think of routines like a comforting rhythm that helps keep things on track. Having regular times for meals, medication, and activities can create a sense of stability and ease any confusion or anxiety.

2.Break Tasks into Smaller Steps: Imagine breaking down a big task into smaller pieces, like solving a puzzle one piece at a time. This makes tasks easier to understand and complete, reducing frustration and making success more achievable.

3.Choose Meaningful Activities: Just like picking your favorite game to play, choose activities that are meaningful and enjoyable for the person with dementia. Whether it's gardening, listening to music, or flipping through old photo albums, activities that hold personal meaning can bring joy and purpose.

4.Adjust Activities to Abilities: As dementia progresses, certain activities might become more challenging. That's okay! Modify activities to match the person's abilities, making them easier to participate in and enjoy. Simplify games or crafts, offer helpful hints, and focus on what the person can still do well.

5. Encourage Independence:

Everyone likes to feel in control of their day. Encourage the person with dementia to make their own choices whenever possible, like deciding what to wear or what activity to do next. This helps them feel empowered and respected.

6. Offer Support When Needed: Sometimes, a little help goes a long way. Be there to lend a hand or offer guidance during activities, but let the person take the lead as much as they can. It's all about finding the right balance between independence and assistance.

7. Create a Safe Space: Just like setting up a game area, create a safe and supportive environment for the person with dementia. Remove any hazards or obstacles, and make adjustments to support their mobility and comfort. Visual cues, like signs or labels, can also help them navigate their surroundings.

8.Stay Patient and Flexible: Remember, every day is different. Be patient and flexible, adapting plans and activities as needed. Some days might be smoother than others, but with a positive attitude and a willingness to adjust, you can make each day the best it can be.

In short, adapting daily routines and activities for someone with dementia is all about making each day as enjoyable and manageable as possible. By keeping things simple, meaningful, and tailored to the person's abilities, you can create a positive and supportive environment where they can thrive.

Chapter 2

Treatment Options and Relief Strategies

Herbal Remedies and Supplements

When it comes to dementia, some people turn to herbal remedies and supplements as an alternative or addition to traditional medications. These natural options have caught attention for their potential benefits, but it's crucial to understand them properly and talk to a healthcare provider before trying them out.

One popular herb people look at is Ginkgo biloba. It comes from the leaves of the Ginkgo tree and is believed to improve memory and cognitive function in people with dementia. However, studies have shown mixed results, so more research is needed to know for sure.

Another herb is Huperzine A, extracted from a type of club moss. It's thought to work similarly to prescription medications by helping with memory and learning. While some studies look promising, we still need more research to make sure it's safe and effective in the long run.

Curcumin is a compound found in turmeric, a spice. It has antioxidant and anti-inflammatory properties, which might help protect brain cells from damage and reduce inflammation linked to dementia. While early studies show some potential, we need more evidence to be sure.

Omega-3 fatty acids, found in fish oil supplements, are also being studied. They're essential for brain health and may improve cognitive function and reduce the risk of cognitive decline in older adults. But again, more research is needed to confirm these findings.

Other natural compounds like vitamin E, vitamin B12, and ginseng are also being looked at. Vitamin E is an antioxidant that might protect brain cells, while vitamin B12 is vital for brain health and function. Ginseng, an herb used in traditional medicine, could also improve memory and cognitive function.

Before trying any herbal remedy or supplement, it's crucial to talk to a healthcare provider, especially if you're taking other medications or have health conditions. These natural options aren't regulated like prescription drugs, so their safety and effectiveness can vary. Plus, a healthcare provider can offer personalized advice and keep an eye out for any side effects or interactions.

Exploring Natural Remedies for Dementia Symptoms

Dementia is a big challenge, but there are natural ways to help manage its symptoms and make life a bit easier. Here are some simple ideas:

1.Stay Active: Exercise isn't just good for the body—it's great for the brain too! Activities like walking, swimming, or yoga can help keep the brain healthy and improve mood. Plus, they're fun ways to stay active and feel good.

2.Keep Your Brain Busy: Just like muscles, the brain needs regular exercise too! Doing puzzles, reading books, or learning new things can help keep the brain sharp and delay the progression of dementia symptoms. It's like giving your brain a workout!

3.Hang Out with Friends: Socializing with friends and family is super important for staying happy and healthy. Spending time with loved ones, chatting, or playing games together can lift spirits and make each day brighter.

4.Eat Well: A healthy diet is like fuel for the brain. Eating plenty of fruits, veggies, whole grains, and lean proteins can provide essential nutrients that support brain function and overall well-being. Plus, it's tasty and good for the body too!

5.Try Herbal Remedies: Some herbs and supplements, like Ginkgo biloba, have been studied for their potential benefits in dementia. While more research is needed, some people find them helpful in managing symptoms. Just be sure to talk to a healthcare provider before trying any new supplements.

6.Enjoy Aromatherapy: Aromatherapy can be a soothing way to relax and unwind. Certain scents, like lavender or rosemary, may help reduce stress, improve sleep, and boost overall well-being. It's like giving yourself a mini spa day at home!

7.Listen to Music: Music has a special way of touching our hearts and minds. Listening to favorite songs or playing instruments can stimulate the brain, reduce anxiety, and bring joy to individuals with dementia. It's a beautiful way to connect with emotions and memories.

8.Practice Relaxation Techniques: Taking time to relax and unwind is important for everyone, especially those living with dementia. Practices like meditation, deep breathing, or yoga can help reduce stress and improve overall well-being. It's like giving your mind a little vacation!

While these natural remedies can be helpful, it's important to talk to a healthcare provider before trying anything new. They can offer personalized advice and make sure it's safe for you or your loved one. With the right support and guidance, natural remedies can be a valuable addition to managing dementia symptoms and improving quality of life.

Herbal Supplements and Their Potential Benefits

Dementia is tough, but some herbal supplements have been looked at to see if they can help manage its symptoms and make life easier for those affected.

1. Ginkgo Biloba: This supplement comes from the leaves of the Ginkgo tree. It's been used for a long time in traditional medicine and is thought to help with memory and thinking. Some studies suggest it might improve cognitive function in people with dementia, especially Alzheimer's disease. But not all studies agree, so more research is needed to be sure.

2.Huperzine A: This supplement is made from a type of club moss. It's believed to work like prescription medications for dementia by protecting brain cells involved in memory and learning. Some studies show it might improve cognitive function and memory in people with dementia, but we need more research to know for sure if it's safe and effective.

3.Curcumin: Found in the spice turmeric, curcumin has antioxidant and anti-inflammatory properties. Some studies suggest it might protect brain cells from damage and reduce inflammation related to dementia. Early research looks promising, but more studies are needed to confirm its benefits.

4.Omega-3 Fatty Acids: These are healthy fats found in fish oil supplements. They're important for brain health and may improve cognitive function and reduce the risk of cognitive decline in older adults. However, more research is needed to know how much and how long to take them for the best results.

While these herbal supplements show potential, it's crucial to be cautious and talk to a healthcare provider before trying them. Herbal supplements aren't regulated like prescription drugs, so their safety and effectiveness can vary. Plus, they might interact with other medications or health conditions, so it's important to get expert advice.

In summary, herbal supplements like Ginkgo biloba, Huperzine A, curcumin, and omega-3 fatty acids have been studied for their potential benefits in managing dementia symptoms. While some studies look promising, more research is needed to confirm their effectiveness and safety. Always talk to a healthcare provider before trying any new supplements, and remember that they should be part of a comprehensive treatment plan for dementia.

Safety Considerations and Potential Interactions

When it comes to taking care of someone with dementia, safety is super important. People with dementia might forget things or get confused, which can put them at risk of accidents or problems with their medications. Here's what caregivers need to know to keep their loved ones safe:

1.Make the Environment Safe: It's essential to remove any hazards around the house that could cause accidents. Simple things like adding grab bars in the bathroom or clearing clutter from walkways can help prevent falls. Using locks on doors and windows can also stop them from wandering away and getting lost.

2.Manage Medications Carefully: Many people with dementia take several medications to stay healthy. But taking too many or mixing them up can be dangerous. Caregivers should keep track of all the medications their loved one takes and let their healthcare provider know about any changes. It's essential to watch out for any side effects or problems with the medications.

3.Watch Out for Interactions: Some medications can interact with each other or with other things like alcohol or herbal supplements. These interactions can make problems worse, so it's crucial to be careful. Caregivers should learn about potential interactions and talk to their healthcare provider before trying anything new.

4.Prevent Accidents at Home: People with dementia might forget how to do things safely, so it's essential to make the home as accident-proof as possible. That means locking away things like cleaning supplies or sharp objects, and using safety devices like stove guards or smoke detectors to keep them safe.

5.Be Mindful of Environmental Factors: Sometimes, things like extreme temperatures can be dangerous for people with dementia because they might not realize when it's too hot or too cold. Caregivers should keep an eye on the environment and make sure their loved ones are comfortable and safe.

By taking these steps to ensure safety and avoid interactions, caregivers can help keep their loved ones with dementia safe and comfortable at home. It's essential to stay vigilant and seek help from healthcare providers whenever needed to provide the best possible care.

Chapter 3
Dietary Interventions

The Role of Nutrition in Dementia Management

Food is not just about filling our bellies, it is also crucial for keeping our brains and bodies healthy, especially for those dealing with dementia. Here's why:

1. Keeping the Brain Happy: Just like our muscles need the right fuel to work well, our brains need the right nutrients too. Things like omega-3 fatty acids, found in fish, nuts, and seeds, and antioxidants, found in fruits and veggies, help protect our brains from damage and keep them sharp.

2. Staying Strong and Healthy: Eating a balanced diet isn't just good for the brain—it's good for the

whole body too. Without the right nutrients, people with dementia can lose weight, become malnourished, and face other health problems that make their dementia worse.

3. Feeding Good Moods: Have you ever felt grumpy when you're hungry? Imagine feeling like that all the time! Eating well can help stabilize moods and keep people with dementia feeling happier and more relaxed.

4. Drinking Enough: Staying hydrated is super important for everyone, but especially for people with dementia. If they don't drink enough, they can feel confused, dizzy, or even sick. Caregivers need to make sure their loved ones are drinking plenty of fluids throughout the day.

5. Making Mealtime Easy: Sometimes, people with dementia have trouble eating or swallowing. Caregivers can help by making sure food is easy to eat, cutting it into small pieces, or even helping with feeding if necessary.

6. Creating a Nice Meal Atmosphere: Mealtime should be a pleasant experience, free from stress and distractions. Caregivers can make it more

enjoyable by setting a regular meal schedule, serving tasty and nutritious foods, and making mealtimes social and fun.

7.Respecting Tastes and Traditions: Everyone has foods they like and foods they don't. Caregivers should try to serve foods that their loved ones enjoy and respect any cultural or dietary preferences they have.

By paying attention to what they eat and making sure they're getting the right nutrients, people with dementia can stay healthier and happier for longer. Caregivers play a big role in making sure their loved ones are eating well and feeling their best, so it's essential to take food seriously when managing dementia.

Foods and Nutrients That Support Cognitive Health

When someone has dementia, their brain needs extra care. Eating the right foods can help keep their brain working as well as possible. Here are some tasty foods that can give their brain a boost:

1. Fatty Fish: Fish like salmon, trout, and sardines are super rich in omega-3 fatty acids. These healthy fats are like brain fuel and can help keep their thinking sharp.

2. Berries : Who doesn't love berries? Blueberries, strawberries, and raspberries are full of antioxidants that protect the brain from damage and keep it working well.

3. Leafy Greens: Spinach, kale, and Swiss chard might not be everyone's favorite, but they're excellent for the brain. They're packed with vitamins and minerals that help keep the brain healthy.

4. Nuts and Seeds: Walnuts, almonds, and seeds like flaxseeds and chia seeds are like little brain boosters. They're full of healthy fats, protein, and antioxidants that keep the brain in top shape.

5. Whole Grains: Foods like oats, brown rice, and quinoa are whole grains that give the brain a steady supply of energy. They're like a power-up for thinking and memory.

6. Turmeric: This spice contains something called curcumin, which is great for the brain. It fights off

damage and can help improve memory and thinking skills.

7.Dark Chocolate: Yes, you read that right—dark chocolate! It's full of antioxidants that keep the brain healthy. Just remember, moderation is key!

8.Coffee and Tea: A cup of coffee or tea can be like a little pick-me-up for the brain. They have caffeine and antioxidants that can help improve alertness and thinking skills.

By adding these yummy foods to their diet, people with dementia can give their brain the extra boost it needs to stay sharp and healthy. Plus, they're delicious too!

Developing a Dementia-Friendly Diet Plan

When making a diet plan for someone with dementia, it's essential to choose foods that are good for their brain, easy to eat, and match their likes and needs. Here's how to do it in a way that's easy to understand:

1.Pick Healthy Foods: Choose foods that help their brain work well, like fruits, veggies, whole grains, lean meats, and good fats. These foods have vitamins and stuff that keep the brain healthy.

2.Get Lots of Colors and Textures: Use lots of colorful fruits and veggies—they're not just pretty; they're full of good stuff for the brain. Also, mix up the textures of food to make eating more interesting.

3.Eat Often, but Little: Instead of three big meals, have lots of small meals and snacks throughout the day. It's easier to eat that way, and it keeps the brain fueled up.

4.Drink Plenty of Water: Drinking enough water is super important for everyone, especially for people with dementia. Offer water, tea, or juicy fruits to keep them hydrated.

5.Stay Away from Junk Food: Try to avoid sugary snacks and processed foods. They don't help the brain and can make things worse. Stick to real, healthy food instead.

6.Respect Their Tastes and Traditions: Serve foods they like and are used to eating. Everyone has foods they love, and it's essential to keep those in the diet plan.

7.Make Food Easy to Eat: Sometimes, eating can be hard for people with dementia. Make sure the food is soft or cut into small pieces to make it easier to chew and swallow.

8.Eat Together and Have Fun: Mealtime should be fun and social. Sit down together, talk, and enjoy the food. It's not just about eating; it's about spending time together.

9.Check-in and Make Changes: Keep an eye on how they're eating and feeling. If something's not working, change it up. And don't be afraid to ask for help from a doctor or dietitian.

By making a diet plan that's good for their brain, easy to eat, and enjoyable, you can help someone with dementia stay healthy and happy. It's all about making sure they get the right food in a way that works for them.

Chapter 4

Physical Activity and Exercise

Exercise as a Non-Pharmacological Treatment for Dementia

Medication is not the only answer for managing dementia. Exercise is a fantastic non-drug treatment that can make a big difference in how someone with dementia feels and functions. Here's why:

1. Gets the Body Moving: Exercise is awesome for keeping the body healthy. It strengthens muscles, helps the heart, and improves balance and coordination. For people with dementia, staying active can help them move around better, prevent falls, and keep their bodies strong.

2. Boosts Brain Power: Exercise isn't just good for muscles; it's great for the brain too! When we exercise, our brains release chemicals that help build new brain cells and connections. This can slow down how fast dementia gets worse and even help keep memory and thinking skills sharper.

3.Lifts the Spirits: Ever feel happy and energized after a workout? That's because exercise releases chemicals in the brain that make us feel good. For people with dementia, exercise can help them feel less sad, worried, or upset. It's like a mood booster!

4.Helps Sleep Better: Sleep can be tricky for people with dementia, but exercise can help. When we're active during the day, it's easier to fall asleep at night and stay asleep. Better sleep means more energy and feeling better during the day.

5.Brings People Together: Exercise isn't just something you do alone—it's also a chance to hang out with others. Joining a walking group or exercise class is a fun way for people with dementia to make friends and stay connected. Plus, it's good for the brain to be social!

6.Supports Caregivers Too: Taking care of someone with dementia can be tough, but exercise can help caregivers too. Doing activities together can strengthen their bond, give them a break from stress, and keep them healthy and happy.

Overall, exercise is a super powerful way to help people with dementia feel better, think clearer, and live happier lives. Whether it's going for a walk, dancing, or playing a game, staying active is a great way to make a positive difference for someone with dementia.

Crafting a Diet Plan for Someone with Dementia

Making a diet plan for someone with dementia is all about picking foods that are good for their brain, easy to eat, and match their likes and needs. Here's how to do it in a way that's easy to understand:

1.Start with Healthy Foods: Choose foods that are full of good stuff like fruits, veggies, whole grains, lean meats, and healthy fats. These foods help keep the brain healthy and strong.

2.Get Brain-Boosting Foods: Add foods that are known to help the brain work better, like fatty fish (think salmon and trout), which have omega-3 fatty acids that are super good for the brain.

3.Make Food Easy to Eat: Think about how easy it is for them to chew, swallow, and eat by themselves. Soft foods or things cut into small pieces can make it easier. And don't forget to provide utensils or special tools if they need help eating.

4.Keep Them Hydrated: It's essential to make sure they drink enough water and other liquids throughout the day. Offer things like water, herbal teas, and juicy fruits to keep them hydrated and feeling good.

5.Stay Away from Junk: Try to avoid sugary snacks and processed foods—they don't help the brain and can make things worse. Stick to real, healthy food instead.

6.Respect What They Like to Eat: Serve foods they enjoy and are used to eating. Everyone has foods they love, and it's important to keep those in their diet plan.

7.Stick to a Routine: Having regular meal and snack times can make things easier and less confusing for them. It's nice to have a routine they can count on.

8.Eat Together and Have Fun: Mealtime should be a time to enjoy food and each other's company. Try to sit down together, talk, and make it a positive experience.

9.Keep an Eye on Things: Pay attention to how they're eating and feeling. If something's not working, it's okay to make changes. And don't be afraid to ask for help if you need it.

By making a diet plan that's good for their brain, easy to eat, and enjoyable, you can help someone with dementia stay healthy and happy. It's all about making sure they get the right food in a way that works for them.

Types of Exercises Beneficial for Cognitive Function

When it comes to keeping the brain in shape for people with dementia, exercise is like magic! Here are some fun types of exercises that can help:

1.Walking and Jogging: Going for a walk or jog gets the heart pumping and brings more blood to the brain. It's like giving the brain a big hug! Walking or jogging for about 30 minutes a day can help improve memory and thinking skills.

2.Lifting Weights: Lifting weights or using resistance bands makes muscles stronger. But did you know it also helps the brain? It's true! Strength training exercises can help build new brain cells and make connections between them.

3.Yoga and Tai Chi: These are super cool exercises that involve moving your body in different ways while focusing on breathing and balance. They're like a dance for the brain! Yoga and tai chi can help improve memory, reduce stress, and make you feel more calm and focused.

4.Stretching and Flexibility: Stretching exercises, like reaching for the sky or touching your toes, can help keep muscles flexible and joints moving smoothly. It's like giving the body a nice stretch, which also helps the brain feel more relaxed and ready to learn.

5.Mind Games and Puzzles: Games like Sudoku, crossword puzzles, and memory games are like a workout for the brain! They challenge your memory, attention, and problem-solving skills, making the brain stronger and smarter.

6.Dancing: Who doesn't love dancing? It's not just fun; it's also great for the brain! Dancing gets your body moving and your heart pumping, while also challenging your coordination and rhythm. Plus, dancing with friends is a fantastic way to socialize and have a good time.

7.Playing Sports: Whether it's basketball, soccer, or tennis, playing sports is an awesome way to stay active and have fun. Sports help improve coordination, teamwork, and mental focus—all of which are great for the brain!

8.Mindfulness and Meditation: Taking a few minutes each day to practice mindfulness or meditation can help calm the mind and reduce stress. It's like giving the brain a little break from all the busyness of life, allowing it to recharge and reset.

By trying out different types of exercises, you can keep your brain healthy, strong, and ready for anything that comes its way—even dementia! So, grab a friend, put on your sneakers, and get moving!

Implementing an Exercise Routine for Individuals with Dementia

Did you know that doing exercise can be super helpful for people with memory problems like dementia? It can make them feel happier, help them think better, and even make their bodies stronger.

When someone has memory problems, exercise can be like magic for them! It can make them feel less sad or worried, help them remember things better, and even help them sleep better at night. Plus, it can stop them from falling down and keep their hearts healthy. Doing exercise can also give them a special routine, which makes them feel good inside.

Things to Think About When Making Exercise Plans
Okay, so when we make exercise plans for people with memory problems, we need to think about a few things:

1. Everyone is Different: Just like how we all have different favorite foods, people with memory

problems like different kinds of exercise. We need to find out what they like and what they can do easily.

2. Keep it Simple: We need to explain things in an easy way and show them how to do the exercises. It's like teaching someone a new game – we need to make it fun and easy to understand.

3. Safety First: We need to make sure the place where they do exercise is safe, without any things they could trip over. And if they need help walking or holding onto something, we should give them that help.

4. Make it Fun: Exercise doesn't have to be boring! We can do lots of fun things like dancing, walking, or even just stretching. The important thing is to make it enjoyable for them.

5. Friends are Important: Exercising with friends or family can make it even more fun! It's like playing a game together – we can encourage each other and have a good time.

Tips for Making Exercise Plans Fun

Here are some tips to make exercising fun for people with memory problems:

1. Set a Regular Time: Pick a time of day when they feel most awake and ready to have fun.

2. Make a Cool Space: Choose a quiet and comfy place for exercise time. Maybe we can play some nice music and have soft lights to make it cozy.

3. Take it Step by Step: We should show them each exercise slowly and clearly. And if they don't get it at first, that's okay! We can be patient and help them until they feel confident.

4. Be Flexible: Sometimes, they might not feel like exercising, and that's okay too! We can change the plan or take breaks if they need it.

5. Keep Track of Progress: We can celebrate little victories and see how they're getting better at exercise over time. It's like leveling up in a game – every little bit counts!

Conclusion
So, there you have it – exercise can be super fun and helpful for people with memory problems like

dementia. By thinking about what they like, keeping it simple and safe, and having a good time together, we can make exercise a special part of their day that they'll look forward to!

Chapter 5

Mindfulness and Relaxation Techniques

Mind-Body Practices for Stress Reduction and Symptom Management

Living with dementia can be tough, right? But guess what? There are some cool things called mind-body practices that can help make things better. These practices can help reduce stress and make you feel happier overall. Let's dive in and learn more about how they work!

Understanding Mind-Body Practices
Mind-body practices are like superpowers for your mind and body. They include things like mindfulness meditation, yoga, tai chi, and deep breathing exercises. These practices help you relax, calm your mind, and feel more connected to yourself. It's like giving your brain and body a big hug!

Benefits for People with Dementia

So, why are mind-body practices so awesome for people with dementia? Well, they do a bunch of cool things:

1. Stress Reduction: Mind-body practices help you chill out and relax. They can calm your mind and make you feel less stressed, which is super important when you're dealing with dementia.

2. Improved Thinking: Some of these practices can actually help your brain work better! They might help you remember things more easily and think more clearly, which is really helpful when you're trying to do stuff every day.

3. Feeling Happier: Mind-body practices can boost your mood and make you feel happier overall. They can help you feel more peaceful inside and deal with any sad or worried feelings you might have.

4. Better Sleep: Have trouble sleeping? Mind-body practices like meditation can help you relax before bedtime, so you can get a better night's sleep. And we all know how important sleep is for feeling good!

5. Making Friends: When you do these practices in a group, like yoga or tai chi classes, you get to meet new friends and have fun together. It's like joining a cool club where everyone supports each other!

How to Get Started with Mind-Body Practices
Ready to give mind-body practices a try? Here's how to get started:

1. Take it Slow: Start with simple exercises and go at your own pace. There's no rush, so just relax and enjoy the process.

2. Keep it Simple: Choose practices that are easy to understand and don't require a lot of complicated moves. You want to have fun, not get frustrated!

3. Find a Quiet Space: Pick a peaceful spot for your practice, away from distractions and noise. It's easier to relax when you're in a calm environment.

4. Be Kind to Yourself: Remember, it's okay to make mistakes or take breaks. Be patient with yourself and celebrate your progress along the way.

5. Have Fun: Most importantly, have fun with it! Enjoy the feeling of relaxation and connection that comes with mind-body practices.

Mindfulness Meditation and its Impact on Cognitive Function

Dementia encompasses a range of neurodegenerative disorders characterized by progressive cognitive decline, affecting memory, reasoning, and other cognitive functions essential for daily functioning. Alzheimer's disease, vascular dementia, and Lewy body dementia are among the most common forms. As the global population ages, dementia poses significant challenges to healthcare systems and society as a whole, underscoring the urgent need for effective interventions.

The Role of Mindfulness Meditation:
Mindfulness meditation involves cultivating present-moment awareness through focused attention and non-judgmental acceptance of thoughts, sensations, and emotions. By training individuals to engage fully with their experiences, mindfulness practices hold the potential to enhance cognitive functioning and mitigate the symptoms of dementia.

Impact on Cognitive Function:
Research exploring the effects of mindfulness meditation on cognitive function in dementia has yielded promising findings. Studies have reported improvements in attention, memory, and executive functioning among individuals with mild cognitive impairment and early-stage dementia following participation in mindfulness-based interventions. These improvements are attributed to the neuroplasticity of the brain, whereby mindfulness practices promote structural and functional changes that support cognitive resilience and adaptation.

Mechanisms of Action:
Several mechanisms underlie the cognitive benefits of mindfulness meditation in dementia. Firstly, mindfulness practices may enhance cognitive reserve by strengthening neural networks and synaptic connections, thereby offsetting the impact of neurodegenerative processes. Secondly, mindfulness promotes stress reduction and regulates the hypothalamic-pituitary-adrenal (HPA) axis, which plays a key role in modulating cognitive function. By reducing stress levels, mindfulness may mitigate the detrimental effects of chronic stress on the brain and cognition. Moreover,

mindfulness meditation fosters emotional regulation and psychological well-being, which are integral aspects of cognitive health in dementia.

Clinical Implications:
The integration of mindfulness-based interventions into dementia care holds significant promise for improving outcomes and enhancing quality of life for affected individuals and their caregivers. Mindfulness programs tailored to the unique needs and capabilities of individuals with dementia can provide valuable support in managing cognitive symptoms and promoting psychological resilience. Moreover, mindfulness practices may complement existing pharmacological and psychosocial interventions, offering a holistic approach to dementia care.

Challenges and Considerations:
While the potential benefits of mindfulness meditation in dementia are promising, several challenges warrant consideration. Adaptations may be necessary to accommodate the cognitive and sensory impairments common in individuals with advanced dementia. Furthermore, the accessibility and scalability of mindfulness programs in healthcare settings require careful attention to

ensure widespread implementation and equitable access for diverse populations. Future research should continue to explore the optimal delivery formats, duration, and dosage of mindfulness interventions for maximum efficacy in dementia care.

Incorporating Relaxation Techniques into Daily Care

Caring for someone with dementia can be emotionally and physically demanding, both for the caregiver and the individual with dementia. Integrating relaxation techniques into daily care routines can significantly benefit both parties, reducing stress, improving mood, and enhancing overall well-being. Here are some practical ways to incorporate relaxation techniques into the daily care of someone with dementia:

1.Mindfulness Meditation: Encourage moments of mindfulness throughout the day. Simple practices like deep breathing exercises or guided meditation can help reduce anxiety and promote relaxation. Find a quiet space and gently guide the individual through a short meditation session, focusing on the present moment and sensations within the body.

2.Music Therapy: Music has a powerful effect on mood and cognition. Create playlists of familiar and soothing music that the individual enjoys. Play the music during daily activities such as mealtime, bathing, or before bedtime. Music can evoke positive emotions, reduce agitation, and improve overall quality of life for individuals with dementia.

3.Gentle Exercise: Engage in gentle exercises tailored to the individual's abilities. Activities like walking, tai chi, or chair yoga can help reduce stress and promote relaxation. Incorporate these exercises into daily routines, making them enjoyable and accessible for the person with dementia.

4.Aromatherapy: Explore the use of essential oils to create a calming atmosphere. Lavender, chamomile, and rosemary are known for their relaxing properties. Diffuse these oils in the living space or apply diluted oils to pulse points for a soothing effect. Be mindful of any allergies or sensitivities the individual may have.

5.Nature Therapy: Spending time outdoors can have therapeutic benefits for individuals with dementia. Take leisurely walks in a garden or park, allowing the person to connect with nature and enjoy the sights and sounds of the outdoors. Nature therapy can reduce stress, improve mood, and enhance overall well-being.

6.Art and Creativity: Engage in creative activities that promote relaxation and self-expression. Provide opportunities for drawing, painting, or crafting activities that cater to the individual's interests and abilities. Art therapy can be a valuable tool for reducing anxiety and promoting a sense of accomplishment and joy.

7.Massage Therapy: Gentle touch can be incredibly soothing for individuals with dementia. Offer gentle massages using lotion or oils, focusing on areas of tension and discomfort. Massage therapy can promote relaxation, improve circulation, and enhance the bond between caregiver and recipient.

8.Reminiscence Therapy: Reminiscing about past experiences can evoke positive emotions and reduce stress. Look through photo albums, listen to familiar stories, or engage in activities that bring back happy memories. Reminiscence therapy can help individuals with dementia feel validated, understood, and connected to their personal history.

9.Breathing Exercises: Teach simple breathing techniques to promote relaxation and reduce anxiety. Encourage slow, deep breaths, inhaling through the nose and exhaling through the mouth. Practice these breathing exercises together during moments of stress or agitation to help the individual regain a sense of calmness and control.

10.Sensory Stimulation: Explore sensory activities that engage the senses and promote relaxation. Provide textured objects to touch, soothing music to listen to, or scented items to smell. Sensory stimulation can help individuals with dementia feel grounded, calm, and more present in the moment.

Incorporating relaxation techniques into daily care routines for individuals with dementia requires patience, creativity, and flexibility. It's essential to observe the individual's preferences and responses, adapting activities accordingly to ensure maximum comfort and enjoyment. By prioritizing relaxation and well-being, caregivers can create a supportive environment that promotes a sense of peace and dignity for those living with dementia

Chapter 6

Cognitive Stimulation Activities

Engaging Activities to Support Brain Health and Function

Living with dementia doesn't mean the fun has to stop! Engaging in activities that stimulate the brain can be incredibly beneficial for individuals with dementia. These activities not only provide enjoyment and a sense of purpose but also help maintain cognitive function and slow down the progression of the disease. Let's explore some fun and engaging activities that support brain health in dementia.

1. Memory Games and Puzzles
Memory games and puzzles are excellent for exercising the brain and keeping it sharp. Activities like crossword puzzles, Sudoku, word searches, and memory matching games can help improve memory, concentration, and problem-solving skills. These games can be adapted to suit different levels

of ability, making them accessible and enjoyable for individuals with dementia.

2. Creative Arts and Crafts

Engaging in creative arts and crafts activities can stimulate the brain and provide a sense of accomplishment. Painting, drawing, coloring, and crafting with clay or paper are great ways to express creativity and engage the senses. These activities can also promote relaxation and reduce stress, contributing to overall well-being.

3. Music and Dance

Music has a powerful effect on the brain and can evoke memories and emotions in individuals with dementia. Listening to familiar songs, singing, or playing musical instruments can be incredibly therapeutic. Similarly, dancing is a fun and enjoyable way to engage the body and mind, promoting physical activity and social interaction.

4. Gardening and Nature Activities

Spending time outdoors and engaging in gardening activities can have a positive impact on brain health. Gardening allows individuals to connect with nature, engage their senses, and experience a sense of accomplishment as they nurture plants and flowers.

Simple tasks like planting seeds, watering plants, or tending to a small garden can provide both physical and cognitive benefits.

5. Storytelling and Reminiscence

Sharing stories and reminiscing about past experiences can stimulate the brain and promote social interaction. Encourage individuals with dementia to share memories, anecdotes, and personal stories with others. This can be done through group discussions, storytelling sessions, or memory books filled with photos and mementos. Reminiscing about the past can help individuals feel connected and valued, fostering a sense of belonging and identity.

6. Physical Exercise and Movement

Physical exercise is not only important for maintaining physical health but also for supporting brain function. Activities like walking, gentle stretching, chair exercises, and yoga can improve circulation, reduce stress, and enhance mood. Regular exercise also promotes the release of endorphins, which are natural mood boosters that can help alleviate symptoms of depression and anxiety.

7. Mindfulness and Meditation

Practicing mindfulness and meditation can help calm the mind, reduce stress, and improve overall well-being. Simple breathing exercises, guided meditation sessions, and mindfulness practices can be beneficial for individuals with dementia. These activities encourage relaxation, focus, and present-moment awareness, providing a sense of peace and tranquility amidst the challenges of dementia.

Conclusion

Engaging in activities that support brain health is essential for individuals living with dementia. Whether it's playing memory games, creating art, listening to music, or spending time outdoors, there are countless ways to stimulate the mind and promote overall well-being. By incorporating these activities into daily routines, individuals with dementia can enjoy a higher quality of life and maintain cognitive function for as long as possible.

Cognitive Stimulation Therapy Approaches

Cognitive Stimulation Therapy (CST) is a non-pharmacological intervention specifically designed to support individuals with dementia by providing structured and stimulating activities. CST approaches aim to engage cognitive functions, enhance social interaction, and improve overall well-being. Here's a detailed exploration of CST approaches and their benefits for individuals living with dementia:

1. Structured Group Sessions:
   CST typically involves structured group sessions led by trained facilitators. These sessions often take place in a supportive and inclusive environment, such as a community center or care facility. Group settings encourage social interaction, promote a sense of belonging, and provide opportunities for individuals with dementia to engage with others in meaningful activities.

2. Multisensory Stimulation:
   CST activities often incorporate multisensory stimulation to engage various cognitive functions and sensory modalities. Visual, auditory, tactile, and olfactory stimuli can be utilized to create a rich and immersive experience. For example, reminiscence activities may involve looking at old photographs,

listening to music from different eras, or handling familiar objects related to past experiences.

3. Cognitive Exercises:

CST includes a variety of cognitive exercises designed to stimulate different aspects of cognition, such as memory, attention, language, and executive function. These exercises may include word games, puzzles, storytelling, and problem-solving tasks. By challenging cognitive abilities in a supportive and structured environment, individuals with dementia can maintain cognitive function and delay further decline.

4. Reminiscence Therapy:

Reminiscence therapy is a key component of CST, allowing individuals with dementia to recall and share memories from their past. Reminiscence activities may involve group discussions, storytelling, or looking through memory aids such as photo albums or memory boxes. By tapping into long-term memories, reminiscence therapy promotes a sense of continuity, identity, and emotional well-being.

5. Reality Orientation:

Reality orientation techniques are often integrated into CST to help individuals with dementia maintain a connection to their surroundings and temporal context. Facilitators may provide orientation cues, such as calendars, clocks, or visual aids, to help individuals orient themselves to the present time and place. Reality orientation fosters a sense of security and reduces disorientation and confusion.

6. Creative Expression:

CST encourages creative expression through various artistic and expressive activities, such as music, art, drama, and poetry. These activities provide individuals with dementia an outlet for self-expression, communication, and emotional release. Creative expression can also stimulate cognitive function, enhance mood, and promote a sense of accomplishment and self-worth.

7. Validation Therapy:

Validation therapy principles are often applied in CST sessions to acknowledge and validate individuals' emotions, experiences, and perspectives. Facilitators demonstrate empathy, active listening, and nonjudgmental acceptance, creating a supportive and validating environment for individuals with dementia to express themselves freely. Validation therapy fosters trust, emotional connection, and a sense of dignity and respect.

8. Person-Centered Approach:
CST adopts a person-centered approach that respects individuals' preferences, abilities, and unique life experiences. Activities are tailored to match participants' interests, cultural background, and cognitive abilities, ensuring maximum engagement and enjoyment. Facilitators collaborate with individuals with dementia and their caregivers to design personalized CST interventions that meet their specific needs and goals.

Benefits of CST:
Cognitive Stimulation Therapy approaches offer numerous benefits for individuals with dementia, including:
- Improved cognitive function and memory retention
- Enhanced social interaction and communication skills
- Reduced feelings of isolation, loneliness, and depression
- Increased self-esteem, confidence, and sense of purpose

- Enhanced quality of life for individuals with dementia and their caregivers

Creating Stimulating Environments for Individuals with Dementia

Creating stimulating environments for individuals with dementia is essential for promoting cognitive function, emotional well-being, and overall quality of life. These environments should be designed to engage the senses, support independence, and foster a sense of familiarity and security. Here's a comprehensive exploration of strategies for creating stimulating environments for individuals with dementia:

1. Sensory Stimulation:
   Sensory stimulation plays a crucial role in creating stimulating environments for individuals with dementia. Consider incorporating elements that engage multiple senses, such as soothing music, pleasant scents, tactile materials, and visually appealing decor. Sensory-rich environments can

evoke positive emotions, reduce agitation, and enhance overall well-being.

2. Familiarity and Routine:
Individuals with dementia often find comfort and security in familiar surroundings and routines. Create environments that incorporate familiar objects, colors, and layouts to promote a sense of continuity and reduce disorientation. Establishing consistent daily routines can also provide structure and predictability, helping individuals with dementia feel more secure and oriented.

3. Safety and Accessibility:
Safety and accessibility are paramount when designing environments for individuals with dementia. Ensure that spaces are free of hazards and obstacles, with clear pathways and adequate lighting to prevent falls and accidents. Consider implementing safety features such as handrails, grab bars, and non-slip flooring to support mobility and independence.

4. Memory Aids and Reminders:
Incorporate memory aids and reminders throughout the environment to support cognitive function and memory retention. Use visual cues

such as signs, labels, and picture prompts to help individuals navigate their surroundings and remember important information. Memory aids can also include calendars, clocks, and personalized memory books to reinforce temporal orientation and daily routines.

5. Access to Nature and Outdoor Spaces:
Access to nature and outdoor spaces can have significant benefits for individuals with dementia, promoting relaxation, sensory stimulation, and social interaction. Design outdoor areas with comfortable seating, sensory gardens, and walking paths to encourage individuals to spend time outdoors and engage with nature. Natural elements such as plants, flowers, and water features can create a calming and therapeutic environment.

6. Social Engagement and Interaction:
Social engagement is essential for maintaining cognitive function and emotional well-being in individuals with dementia. Design environments that facilitate social interaction and meaningful engagement with others. Common areas with comfortable seating, communal dining spaces, and designated activity areas can encourage

socialization and foster a sense of community among residents.

7. Personalized Spaces:
   Personalization is key to creating stimulating environments for individuals with dementia. Allow residents to personalize their living spaces with familiar belongings, photographs, and mementos that hold sentimental value. Personalized spaces help individuals maintain a sense of identity, autonomy, and connection to their past, enhancing overall well-being.

8. Multi-Sensory Rooms:
   Multi-sensory rooms offer immersive environments designed to stimulate the senses and promote relaxation and engagement. These rooms may feature interactive light displays, soothing sounds, tactile surfaces, and aromatherapy elements. Multi-sensory experiences can help individuals with dementia regulate emotions, reduce stress, and enhance sensory awareness.

9. Flexibility and Adaptability:
   Flexibility and adaptability are essential when designing environments for individuals with dementia. Spaces should be designed to

accommodate changing needs and abilities, with adjustable furniture, modular layouts, and flexible activity spaces. Incorporating versatile design elements allows environments to evolve over time to meet the diverse needs of residents.

10. Staff Training and Support:

Finally, providing ongoing training and support for staff members is crucial for maintaining stimulating environments for individuals with dementia. Educate staff on dementia care best practices, communication techniques, and person-centered approaches to support residents' well-being and quality of life. Encourage staff to engage with residents in meaningful activities and interactions, fostering a positive and supportive care environment.

Chapter 7

Understanding Common Symptoms of Dementia

Memory Loss and Cognitive Decline

Memory loss and cognitive decline in dementia represent a complex and challenging aspect of neurological disorders that profoundly impact individuals, families, and societies. Dementia refers to a group of conditions characterized by progressive impairment in cognitive function, including memory, language, problem-solving, and attention. Alzheimer's disease is the most common form of dementia, but there are several other types, such as vascular dementia, Lewy body dementia, and frontotemporal dementia.

One of the hallmark features of dementia is memory loss. It often begins subtly, with individuals experiencing difficulty remembering recent events or conversations. As the condition progresses, this memory impairment becomes more pronounced, affecting not only short-term memory but also long-term memory. People with dementia may struggle to recall significant life events, names of family members, or even basic personal information.

The cognitive decline associated with dementia extends beyond memory loss. Individuals may experience difficulties in language, including finding the right words, understanding speech, or following conversations. They may also struggle with executive functions, such as planning, organizing, and making decisions. Simple tasks that were once routine become increasingly challenging, leading to frustration and loss of independence.

The underlying mechanisms of memory loss and cognitive decline in dementia are complex and multifaceted. In Alzheimer's disease, for example, the accumulation of abnormal proteins in the brain, such as beta-amyloid plaques and tau tangles, disrupts communication between nerve cells and ultimately leads to cell death. This neuronal damage primarily affects regions of the brain involved in memory and learning, such as the hippocampus and the entorhinal cortex.

In vascular dementia, on the other hand, cognitive decline is often the result of impaired blood flow to the brain due to conditions like stroke or small vessel disease. These disruptions in blood flow can lead to the death of brain cells, resulting in cognitive deficits that may manifest differently from those seen in Alzheimer's disease.

While age is the most significant risk factor for dementia, other factors such as genetics, lifestyle, and comorbidities also play a role. For example, individuals with a family history of dementia are at a higher risk of developing the condition themselves. Additionally, chronic conditions like diabetes, hypertension, and obesity can increase the likelihood of developing vascular dementia.

Diagnosis of dementia typically involves a comprehensive assessment of cognitive function, including memory, language, visuospatial skills, and executive function. Medical professionals may use a combination of neuropsychological tests, brain imaging, and laboratory tests to evaluate cognitive abilities and rule out other possible causes of cognitive impairment.

Unfortunately, there is currently no cure for dementia, and available treatments aim to manage symptoms and slow disease progression. Medications such as cholinesterase inhibitors and memantine may help improve cognitive function and alleviate some symptoms, but their efficacy varies from person to person.

In addition to pharmacological interventions, non-pharmacological approaches such as cognitive stimulation therapy, reminiscence therapy, and physical exercise have shown promise in improving cognitive function and quality of life for individuals with dementia.

Despite ongoing research efforts, dementia remains a significant public health challenge with profound social and economic implications. As the global population continues to age, the prevalence of dementia is expected to rise, underscoring the urgent need for innovative approaches to prevention, diagnosis, and treatment. Addressing memory loss and cognitive decline in dementia requires a multi-faceted approach that encompasses medical, social, and environmental factors to support individuals affected by this devastating condition.

Behavioral and Psychological Symptoms

Behavioral and psychological symptoms in dementia (BPSD) are things that happen to people with dementia that aren't just about memory. They can include getting upset easily, feeling sad or worried, seeing or hearing things that are not there, or believing things that are not true. These symptoms can be really tough for the person with dementia and the people taking care of them.

Imagine if someone you knew with dementia suddenly started pacing around, getting angry for no reason, or feeling really sad all the time. That's what some people with dementia experience. It can be scary and confusing for them and for the people around them.

Sometimes, people with dementia might see things that aren't there or believe things that aren't true. For example, they might think someone is trying to hurt them or steal from them, even if it's not true. This can be really distressing for them and hard for others to understand.

Another common problem is feeling like they don't want to do anything or don't care about anything anymore. This can make it hard for them to enjoy activities they used to like or even to take care of themselves.

Sleeping can also become a problem for people with dementia. They might have trouble sleeping at night or feel really sleepy during the day. Some may wander around at night, which can be dangerous.

These behaviors happen because of changes in the brain caused by dementia. It's not just about forgetting things; it's about the brain not working the way it should. Things like stress, changes in routine, or not feeling well can make these behaviors worse.

Taking care of someone with dementia can be really hard, especially when they have these behaviors. Doctors might give them medicine to help, but sometimes it can have side effects. So, doctors and caregivers also try other things, like talking to them calmly, creating a peaceful environment, or doing activities together.

It's important for caregivers to learn about dementia and how to deal with these behaviors. That way, they can help the person with dementia feel more comfortable and safe. With the right support and understanding, we can make life better for people with dementia and those who care for them.

Physical Challenges and Health Considerations

When someone has dementia, it affects not just their memory but also their physical health and ability to take care of themselves. Let's break down some of the physical challenges and health considerations that come with dementia:

1.Mobility Issues: Dementia can make it hard for someone to walk, keep their balance, or move around easily. Their muscles might get weaker, and they might have trouble coordinating their movements. This can increase the risk of falls and injuries, so it's important to make sure their living environment is safe and free from hazards.

2.Nutritional Problems: People with dementia may forget to eat or lose their appetite, leading to weight loss and malnutrition. They might also have trouble swallowing or forget how to use utensils properly, making it harder for them to eat. Ensuring they have regular, nutritious meals and snacks and encouraging them to drink plenty of fluids can help prevent nutritional deficiencies.

3.Personal Hygiene: Remembering to bathe, brush teeth, or go to the bathroom can become challenging for someone with dementia. They might forget how to do these tasks or feel embarrassed about needing help. Caregivers can assist with personal care tasks in a gentle and respectful manner to help maintain their dignity and hygiene.

4. Managing Other Health Conditions: Dementia can complicate the management of other health conditions, such as diabetes, heart disease, or respiratory problems. People with dementia may have difficulty following medical instructions, remembering to take medications, or communicating symptoms to their healthcare providers. Caregivers and healthcare professionals need to work together to ensure that their other health needs are addressed effectively.

5.Medication Management: Keeping track of medications can be challenging for someone with dementia. They may forget to take their pills, take them at the wrong time, or take the wrong dose. Caregivers can help by organizing their medications, providing reminders, and supervising their medication routine to prevent errors and ensure they're getting the right treatment.

6.Regular Medical Check-ups: People with dementia need regular medical check-ups to monitor their overall health and address any emerging issues. Healthcare providers can assess their physical health, monitor changes in their condition, and adjust treatment plans as needed. Regular check-ups also provide an opportunity to discuss any concerns or symptoms they may be experiencing.

By addressing these physical challenges and health considerations, caregivers can help maintain the well-being and quality of life of individuals living with dementia. It's essential to provide support, understanding, and assistance as needed to help them navigate these challenges and stay as healthy and independent as possible.

Chapter 8

Strategies for Managing Symptoms at Home

Creating a Supportive Environment

Creating a supportive environment for someone with dementia means making sure they feel comfortable, safe, and happy in their surroundings. Here are some ways to do that:

1. Safety First: We want to make sure the place they live in is safe for them. That means removing things they might trip over, like rugs or loose cords. We might also put up handrails or grab bars to help them get around safely. It's important to make sure doors and windows are secure to prevent wandering, especially if they get confused easily.

2. Keep Things Familiar: People with dementia feel more at ease when they're surrounded by things they recognize. That could mean having familiar

pictures, furniture, or decorations around the house. These things can help trigger happy memories and make them feel more comfortable.

3.Stick to a Routine: Having a regular routine can be really helpful for someone with dementia. It gives them a sense of structure and predictability, which can reduce anxiety and confusion. So, we try to keep mealtimes, activities, and bedtime consistent every day.

4.Speak Clearly and Simply: When talking to someone with dementia, it's important to speak slowly and clearly. We use simple words and short sentences to make sure they understand us. We also try to use gestures and facial expressions to help get our message across.

5.Encourage Independence: Even though they might need some help, we try to let them do things on their own as much as possible. This could be things like getting dressed, brushing their teeth, or making a snack. It helps them feel more capable and in control of their own life.

6.Fun Activities: Keeping them engaged in activities they enjoy is important for their well-being. It could be anything from painting and puzzles to listening to music or going for a walk. These activities stimulate their mind and keep them entertained.

7.Spending Time Together: Being around other people is really important for someone with dementia. It helps them feel connected and less lonely. So, we make sure they have opportunities to spend time with family, friends, or other people in their community.

8.Be Flexible: Things might not always go as planned, and that's okay. We need to be flexible and adapt to their changing needs and abilities. If something doesn't work, we try something else until we find what works best for them.

9.Support for Caregivers: Taking care of someone with dementia can be tough, so it's important for caregivers to take care of themselves too. That means getting help when needed, taking breaks, and making time for their own well-being.

By creating a supportive environment and following these tips, we can help someone with dementia feel more comfortable and improve their quality of life.

It's all about making them feel loved, understood, and valued.

Practical Tips for Daily Living

Creating a supportive environment for someone with dementia means making sure they feel comfortable, safe, and happy in their surroundings. Here are some ways to do that:

1.Safety First:We want to make sure the place they live in is safe for them. That means removing things they might trip over, like rugs or loose cords. We might also put up handrails or grab bars to help them get around safely. It's important to make sure doors and windows are secure to prevent wandering, especially if they get confused easily.

2.Keep Things Familiar: People with dementia feel more at ease when they're surrounded by things they recognize. That could mean having familiar pictures, furniture, or decorations around the house. These things can help trigger happy memories and make them feel more comfortable.

3.Stick to a Routine: Having a regular routine can be really helpful for someone with dementia. It gives them a sense of structure and predictability, which can reduce anxiety and confusion. So, we try to keep mealtimes, activities, and bedtime consistent every day.

4.Speak Clearly and Simply: When talking to someone with dementia, it's important to speak slowly and clearly. We use simple words and short sentences to make sure they understand us. We also try to use gestures and facial expressions to help get our message across.

5.Encourage Independence:Even though they might need some help, we try to let them do things on their own as much as possible. This could be things like getting dressed, brushing their teeth, or making a snack. It helps them feel more capable and in control of their own life.

6.Fun Activities:Keeping them engaged in activities they enjoy is important for their well-being. It could be anything from painting and puzzles to listening to music or going for a walk. These activities stimulate their mind and keep them entertained.

7.Spending Time Together: Being around other people is really important for someone with dementia. It helps them feel connected and less lonely. So, we make sure they have opportunities to spend time with family, friends, or other people in their community.

8.Be Flexible: Things might not always go as planned, and that's okay. We need to be flexible and adapt to their changing needs and abilities. If something doesn't work, we try something else until we find what works best for them.

9.Support for Caregivers:Taking care of someone with dementia can be tough, so it's important for caregivers to take care of themselves too. That means getting help when needed, taking breaks, and making time for their own well-being.

By creating a supportive environment and following these tips, we can help someone with dementia feel more comfortable and improve their quality of life. It's all about making them feel loved, understood, and valued.

Seeking Professional Assistance and Supportive Services

Seeking professional assistance and accessing supportive services is essential for individuals living with dementia and their caregivers to navigate the challenges associated with the condition effectively. From diagnosis to ongoing care management, various professionals and services play crucial roles in providing comprehensive support and improving the quality of life for those affected by dementia.

1.Medical Evaluation and Diagnosis: The journey often begins with a medical evaluation by a primary care physician or neurologist. If dementia is suspected, further assessment may include cognitive testing, brain imaging, and blood tests to rule out other possible causes of cognitive decline. A timely and accurate diagnosis is essential for initiating appropriate treatment and planning for the future.

2.Dementia Specialists: Depending on the type and stage of dementia, individuals may benefit from the expertise of specialists such as geriatricians, neurologists, psychiatrists, or neuropsychologists.

These professionals can provide specialized assessments, diagnostic clarification, and tailored treatment recommendations to address specific needs and symptoms associated with dementia.

3.Care Coordination and Case Management: Care coordination services help individuals and their families navigate the complex healthcare system and access necessary resources and support services. Case managers or care coordinators can assist with care planning, coordination of medical appointments, referrals to community resources, and advocacy on behalf of the person with dementia and their caregivers.

4.Memory Clinics and Centers of Excellence: Memory clinics and centers of excellence specialize in the diagnosis, treatment, and management of dementia. These multidisciplinary clinics typically offer comprehensive assessments, individualized care plans, education, and support services for individuals with dementia and their families. They often provide access to clinical trials and research opportunities as well.

5.Home Care Services:Home care agencies offer a range of supportive services to help individuals with dementia remain safely in their own homes for as long as possible. Services may include assistance with activities of daily living (ADLs), medication management, meal preparation, companionship, and respite care for family caregivers. Home care providers can customize care plans to meet the unique needs and preferences of each individual.

6.Adult Day Programs:Adult day programs provide supervised daytime care and socialization for individuals with dementia while offering respite for family caregivers. These programs offer a variety of activities, cognitive stimulation, and therapeutic interventions in a safe and supportive environment. They can help delay institutionalization, reduce caregiver stress, and enhance the overall well-being of participants.

7.Residential Care Facilities: As dementia progresses, individuals may require more intensive care and support than can be provided at home. Residential care facilities, such as assisted living communities or memory care units, offer specialized services and a secure environment for individuals with dementia. These facilities provide assistance with ADLs, medication management, meals, and recreational activities tailored to the needs of residents with dementia.

8. Support Groups and Counseling Services: Support groups and counseling services offer emotional support, practical guidance, and education for individuals with dementia and their caregivers. These groups provide opportunities to connect with others who understand the challenges of dementia caregiving, share experiences, and learn coping strategies. Professional counseling can also help individuals and families navigate the emotional impact of dementia and develop effective coping skills.

9. Legal and Financial Planning: Planning for the future is crucial for individuals with dementia and their families. Legal and financial planning services can help navigate legal issues, advance care planning, and establish power of attorney and healthcare directives. Financial advisors can provide guidance on managing finances, accessing benefits, and planning for long-term care needs.

10. End-of-Life Care and Hospice Services: As dementia progresses, individuals and families may face difficult decisions about end-of-life care.

Hospice services offer compassionate care and support for individuals with advanced dementia and their families, focusing on comfort and quality of life. Hospice teams provide symptom management, emotional support, and bereavement services for families during the end-of-life process.

By seeking professional assistance and accessing supportive services, individuals living with dementia and their caregivers can receive the comprehensive care, resources, and support they need to navigate the challenges of dementia and enhance their quality of life. Collaboration between healthcare professionals,community,organizations, and family caregivers is essential for providing holistic and person-centered care throughout the dementia journey.

www.ingramcontent.com/pod-product-compliance
Lightning Source LLC
Chambersburg PA
CBHW070343230526
45471CB00006B/2422